Perfect Health Diet

Eat Right

By Cathy Wilson
Copyright © 2015

Income Disclaimer

This book contains business strategies, marketing methods and other business advice that, regardless of my own results and experience, may not produce the same results (or any results) for you. I make absolutely no guarantee, expressed or implied, that by following the advice below you will make any money or improve current profits, as there are several factors and variables that come into play regarding any given business.

Primarily, results will depend on the nature of the product or business model, the conditions of the marketplace, the experience of the individual, and situations and elements that are beyond your control.

As with any business endeavor, you assume all risk related to investment and money based on your own discretion and at your own potential expense.

Liability Disclaimer

By reading this book, you assume all risks associated with using the advice given below, with a full understanding that you, solely, are responsible for anything that may occur as a result of putting this information into action in any way, and regardless of your interpretation of the advice.

You further agree that our company cannot be held responsible in any way for the success or failure of your business as a result of the information presented in this book. It is your responsibility to conduct your own due diligence regarding the safe and successful operation of your business if you intend to apply any of our information in any way to your business operations.

Terms of Use

You are given a non-transferable, "personal use" license to this book. You cannot distribute it or share it with other individuals.

Also, there are no resale rights or private label rights granted when purchasing this book. In other words, it's for your own personal use only.

Perfect Health Diet

Eat Right

By Cathy Wilson

Table of Contents

Introduction

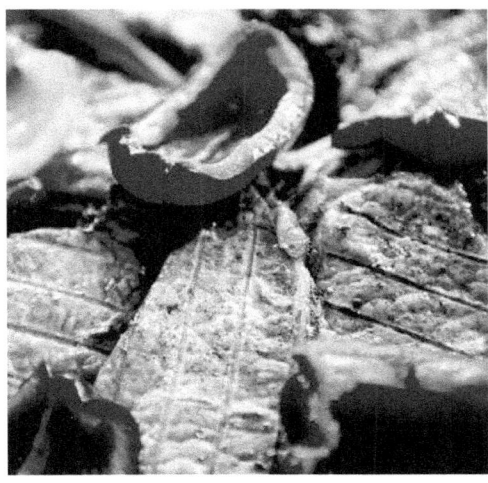

Hi. I am a nutrition expert that has studied and researched eating, fitness, disease, and healthy lifestyle choices for almost twenty years, working closely with fellow nutritionists, specialized doctors, and other health and wellness experts both conventional and holistic and gathering and sort through concepts and beliefs to create practical strategies that will help you get control of your health with a smile.

The Perfect Health Diet is all about back to basics, creating your Perfect Health Diet so you can live a long and productive life. Evolutionary eating, simplistic and natural, nutrient dense, energizing and void of which includes toxic sugars, preservatives and other killer chemicals foreign to our digestive tracts. Toxins contain poison and the key elements summoning free-radicals to invade your body with illness and disease, most debilitating and deadly.

Over time manifesting to slowly steal your quality of life and eventually take it too. The Perfect Health Diet teaches us the importance of listening to our body and fueling it effectively and in the right amounts, regaining trust that must be earned. With healthy, whole natural foods simple and pure, the processed and pumped full of hormones and chemicals, or exposed to harmful environmental toxins.

With The Perfect Health Diet you will lose weight by eating "right," heal chronic disease and deter serious illness from invading. This diet will help you build a body strong and resilient from the inside out. Would you prefer to live in a brick house or a house of straw when the Big Bad Wolf comes huffing and puffing to your door?
It's time to reverse time and not try to reinvent the wheel with regards to eating.

Evolutionary Eating

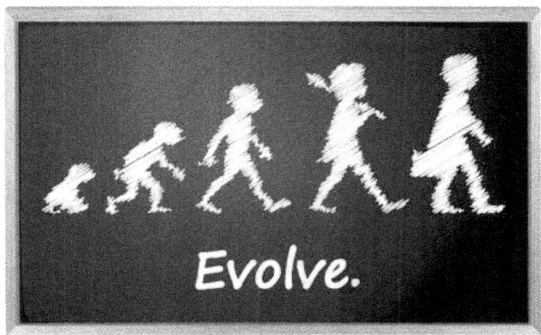

When looking into perfect healthy eating most scientists believe our genetics is where the solution to nutritional eating begins. Evidence shows optimal eating is reflective of the Paleolithic Age, the time of cavemen and dinosaurs, a time where toxic processed and packaged foods didn't exist and strenuous physical labor was required to eat anything. The cycle of tracking, hunting, gathering, cleaning, cooking and feasting was the norm. Feast or famine was reality and sometimes luck dictated whether you lived or died.

Back in time people had no choice but to listen to their body, to work with what mother nature offered and be grateful when there was food available and disease stayed away. Humans had no choice but to accept the harsh realities of life and live reactively. If there was drought and food was scarce people suffered and often perished. They couldn't just stay indoors and look to survive off food from their cupboards and fridges, canned or otherwise. Back in time men, women and children were at the mercy of nature and did their best to survive and thrive.

This concept or train of thought is foreign to us today in our spoiled society. We don't appreciate the conveniences we have and allow greed to get the better of us. Over time we've become lazy and focused on materialistic means, money, fast cars, fancy homes and who has the biggest portfolio. At what price?

It's the biggest price of all. The most valuable asset you have. It's your health. It's time to reprogram our thinking.

Paleolithic Era Expanded
This period lasted about two and a half million years, ending ten thousand years ago when agricultural development commenced. Scientists believe we should learn and open our mind to following in the footstep of these ancient beings in order to get our health back on track.

This hunter-gather cuisine wasn't black and white because people ate what was available. This meant from region to region the meats, berries and plants available to eat changed. So if people got tired of the menu they couldn't just walk down the street to another restaurant.

They had to uproot and brave the weather and other challenges with traveling long distances, in order to relocate anew and begin rebuilding. Learning about what this area of the world offered for food and praying the new spot they picked to live would provide them with a safe haven, void of sickness and disease, with plenty of food to eat with hard work. If there wasn't much game to be hunted the berries and foliage made up the bulk of the diet. People knew how to adapt. Boy do we ever have it easy!

Scientists believe our hunter-gatherer ancestors basically ate a diet with a variety of foods that could be fished and hunted, lots of lean game meats and seafood, along with foods gathered, like nuts, berries, herbs, spices, bugs and plants. This may sound yucky to you but to them it was heaven.

Here lie-in the trouble. In our world today up to SEVENTY percent of the foods we fuel our bodies with today wasn't available to our simplistic nature respecting ancient ancestors. Foods like packaged pastries and cakes, oils, refined sugars, boxed cereals and other fast foods come to mind.

Sure technology seems to control our world today. We want faster, better, more convenient always. Meaning we also want it all and are willing to sacrifice our good health to get it. We don't care that French fries are unhealthy for us because they are fast and taste good. After we make them habit we don't even think about what we are eating or how much, we just keep shoveling them in.

Even in today's world experts still believe if we get rid of all the interference we've created in our lives, remove all the layers of crap we've all got, beneath it all you will find the key to getting healthy. The hunter-gatherer genes are within each one of us and until we recognize this and decide we WANT to change our eating and lifestyle actions for the better. Until we commit to doing whatever it takes to reverse the damage we have caused ourselves and get reacquainted with the simplistic ways of nature. We are just going to keep struggling. Disease and illness is only going to get more aggressive and trigger more interference in the smooth running of our internal. We are literally destroying ourselves from the inside out with progress.

You control you and if you value your life and want at least try to get back perfect health, then you need to open your mind to The Perfect Health Diet and take action. If you want to gain energy, lose fat, deter disease and live happier you need to consider the wise ways of your elders and look into the hunter-gatherer style of eating.

Take from this, what works for you, and start walking in the right direction to perfect health.

Agriculture/Industrial Development Hurting Health?
Next, came the development of agriculture which many experts believe stressed the human body. Foods were introduced that didn't necessarily work in harmony with our body and this minor interference triggered illness and disease, the beginnings of it anyway.

Scientists believed large amounts of milk, grains and domesticated meats were taxing to our system. Just 200 years ago can the Industrial Age where processes furthered. Whole grains and sugars continued to be refined, taking out more of the natural for the price of convenience, cheaper and longer lasting. This "progress" continues today and we live in a society governed by process foods. Everywhere you look you can get convenience that's unhealthy and deadly over time.
Unfortunately most don't seem to care. Do you not value your health and quality of life?

We have progressed so far forward with food that our bodies haven't had the chance to adapt. In other words our food and bodies just don't "fit," healthy or not. Just like trying to fit a square into a circle.
Experts agree we just don't have the physiological ability to absorb the foods we eat and run our bodies optimally. Our "ticking" isn't clicking with the "tocking."

THE CONSEQUENCE?

Sickness, illness, serious disease, minor ailments and weakened bodily systems are the consequences. It's just like filling up your tank with watery gas. Eventually your engine will fail. Causing us to face and deal with obesity, diabetes, heart disease, stroke, cancers, and so many other health ailments WE have created by not taking care of our health. In doing so we are programming our bodies to pass this "factor" along to any children we might have, manifesting the problem instead of changing our behavior to reverse it.

As we continue to feed our bodies unhealthy and unnatural foods, our health problems mount. A cycle of destruction continues. We rely on the medical community to find temporary solutions to the new problems we create. Which themselves cause more problems. Sad but true and the only way we are going to change this pattern is to make a bold move to get to the root of the problem. Experts believe this involves getting back to simple. Paying attention to the hunter-gatherer style of eating and apply these basic principles to our lifestyle, using the knowledge we have gained as a society over time. Using the BEST of both worlds we can create The Perfect Health Diet, but only if you want to.

Western Diet And Ancient Eating Compared
Looking at the way we eat today in general and the strategies of the Paleolithic Era there are obvious differences.

Paleolithic Eating
* Less taxing foods on the kidneys
* Lower glycemic index foods
* Increased fiber
* More vitamins and minerals
* More potassium and less sodium

* Increased lean protein
* Decreased carbohydrates
* More phytochemicals
* Healthy fats only, no Trans fats or overdoses of saturated fats

It really is quite simple and it's humans that make it so confusing. Eating a diet full of natural fresh fruits and vegetables and lean meats, void of processed and packaged unhealthy foods is going to move us as a society towards The Perfect Healthy Diet. The problem with this is we are creatures of habit that don't like change, even for the better.

If you want to get healthy you are going to have to commit to it and stick with it. Change is good but you really do have to WANT it if it's going to happen.

My Thoughts . . .
You have nothing to lose and everything to gain by adapting the ancient methodology of eating. By removing our modern day convenience and looking to eat natural, healthy, chemical free foods that are giving to us by nature, you are choosing to remove the negative interference that is destroying your health today.
Choose taste and convenience, or long health and happiness? The choice is all yours. If you value your health then I will help you get it back.

Breast Milk Just for Babies?

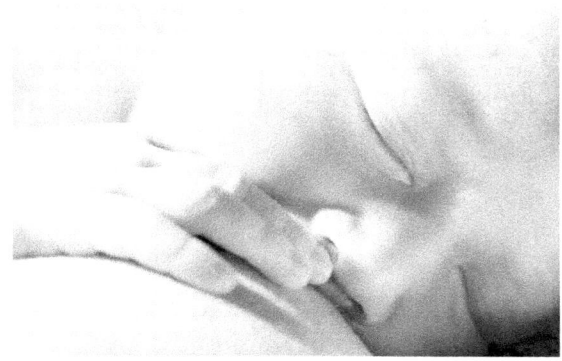

Breast IS best, for babies anyway. As mammals we are born with specific nutritional needs. In fact all mammals can have all their immediate nutritional requirements fulfilled with natures' gift, breast milk.

But is milk best for adults? A question in which there is ample controversy between scientists, experts and professionals.

Milk is simply a whitish liquid created by the mammary or "milk" glands of a mammal. It's the main source of food for baby mammals because they have immature digestive systems and can't breakdown and absorb "adult" food. Milk is easily digestible and provides the perfect mix of vitamins, minerals and protective enzymes to build their body strong.

Think back to your ancestors for years back. If a child didn't have breast milk to drink more often than not they would die of malnutrition. It's a harsh but true reality of the times. Isn't that enough to convince you what mother-nature intended, breast milk, is best?

Experts agree it's the first milk, the yellowish colostrum that gives essential antibodies from the mother to the baby for protection. It's a built-in intrinsic mechanism of nature to increase the chances of survival. Just like handing you a blanket when you are cold, it makes no sense not to use it.

Of course there are exceptions to the rules, but for the most part this makes perfect sense.

Society has conditioned us to think milk is the healthiest drink there is. Fact is experts believe it's either the "perfect" drink or the most dangerous. Young bodies are made for milk, not many are going to argue that. Milk and milk products have also been preached to the younger population for years through the Food Pyramid, taught by nutritionists and through school programs to help children learn healthy eating.

Milk provides foods like butter, kefir, cheese and yogurt, is a good source of protein, calcium and Vitamin D, essential for bone growth and development to start. The flip side of this is lactose intolerance, where the body is unable to breakdown the lactose enzyme. Is this caused from the genetic makeup or is it developed from interference created by the other poor food choices we make, or perhaps the environmental stresses we face daily?

People suffering from lactose intolerance will experience bloating, cramping and loosens bowel movements if they consume lactose foods. The quick fix is taking an oral supplement to replace the missing enzyme.

Milk is the highest reported food allergy. It is also linked to skin conditions like eczema, joint pain, migraine and head pain and sinus issues. There is also the issue of drinking "unhealthy" milk. This includes the dairy milk you purchase from the grocer. This milk is often loaded with growth hormones, pesticides from the contaminated grains and grasses the cows eat, along with antibiotics used to treat disease. Each one of these toxic substances finds its way into the milk you are drinking and contaminates you indirectly.

Does milk really do your body good?

Choosing grass-feed milk is healthier than any others. Some also argue that pasteurization, the process in which store bought milk is heated to "sterilize" it for safe drinking, also destroys the nutritional makeup of the milk. Important protein bonds are lost that make milk more easily digestible for humans.

The problem clearly lies in the delivery of milk to start. Are the hormones found in milk cancer causing? Do they weaken your immune system and stress out your digestion process?

Milk does . . .
* Increase the rate in which you burn body fat
* Help build muscle, bones, skeletal and immune system strength

Facts For Thought - Did you know we are the only mammals that drink milk after being weaned? We're also the only mammals that drink milk provided by other mammals and the only mammals that drink pasteurized milk!

Studies today show the pasteurization process intended to protect our bodies in fact causes issues. It actually forces the bones to lose calcium and causes osteoporosis, bone degeneration, particularly in the elderly.
So where can we get our calcium from? What do cows eat to produce all that milk? They eat plants and grains. Sprouts, nuts, grains, plants and beans are great sources of calcium and protein. Most don't understand this because we've been programmed to believe milk is the end-all-be-all of calcium.

Great Calcium Sources
- Leaf lettuce, beet greens, Swiss chard, collards
- Kale, parsley, mints, broccoli, spouts,
- Clover, lentil, radishes, pumpkin seeds, almonds, sunflower seeds
- Sesame seeds, whole grains
Milk and milk products could do more harm than good. There are a whole lot of foods you can include in your diet instead. Better safe than sorry, don't you think?

My Thinking . . .
You only know what you know and it's tough sometimes to set your personal beliefs aside and look openly and non-judgmentally at the facts to consider. Milk is essential in our lives from birth and evidence shows that as with many things in life we could very well outgrow it. More so, because of all the external factors that will interfere with the quality of the milk and milk products and tax the digestive process. We have created interference with milk and how it benefits our good health. Perhaps it's best to leave it be and use other healthy foods to satiated our need for calcium, Vitamin D and other essential vitamins and minerals milk is able to provide?

Physiology and Diet - The Way We Were Designed to Eat

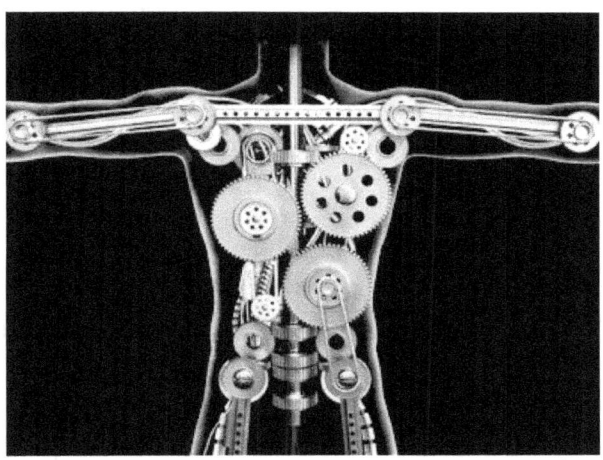

Our ancestors at for more than two and a half million years, we have the same bodies and arguably are designed to eat the same way. The food choices we have just introduced in the past ten thousand years, introducing agriculture, have caused more issues than anything with the function and healthy runny of our internal circuitry.

We have managed to change what we eat, how much and even programmed "when" we eat from listening to our bodies and when they need refueling, in preference of structure and time for social means. We eat high carbohydrate diets (grains, pastries and sweets) foods in huge quantities usually for external reasons, habit, emotions, a daily routine.

Your Body Is Designed To . . .

Eat a diet very high in lean protein, high fat, mod-low carb and nil alcohol. Instead we choose to eat high carbohydrate and low fat which is asking for trouble. Humans are carnivores and should eat more lean meats and supplement with plant products, vegetables and fruits first. We know how our ancestors ate so why would we want to change this or better yet how come we allowed this change? Ancient eating rarely touched grains and definitely didn't have sweets, cakes and pastries regularly.

Eating Rhythm

The problem with eating 5-6 smaller meals a day is you don't give your digestive system a chance to ever relax. This is stressful and taxing on your body as whole. Maybe we do this because of all the sugar we are putting into our system and if we don't eat regularly our blood sugar levels are going to dive bomb?

Eating correctly doesn't take more than 2 meals each day, physiologically speaking, which is exactly how humans ate for more than 2.5 million years! Come on, are you going to argue with that?

They would typically wakeup when their circadian rhythm told them, hunt, cook and eat. They would rest or sleep and repeat the cycle. If they ate twice a day every meal was around 1500 calories, eating three times a day it dropped to 1000 calories.

The benefits of this eating style were rest for the digestive system and the allowance for natural detoxification. It makes sense to me.

Sleep Time

Today we are crazy nut-so! For some reason we think the more productive we are and the less sleep we get the better. Many of us get by on 5-6 hours a night. All this does is it gives us more cycles to eat more crap! Resting less means eating more, less recovery time for your digestive processes and you are going to get fat.

History dictates our ancient friends slept at least 8 hours a night, getting into the rhythm allowed for QUALITY rest that rejuvenated the mind and body EVERY night, not just once on a blue moon.

Calorie Count
Most of us eat WAY too many calories compared to our caloric expenditure, 4-6000 calories per day. Ancient people ate about 3,000 calories per day consistently. Keeping in mind they were much more physically active than we are today. They also listened to their bodies and adjusted when needed. If they happened to strenuously expend more energy on a particular day they would balance things out by eating more, a give take relationship without thought. Back in the day people worked with their body to make sure they provided and never were purposely deprived, a win-win and very forgiving scenario.

Physical Activity
The human body is not meant to vegetate on the couch 24/7, but it's also not designed to work out intensely more than 2-3 times a week. We have to work at this and make time specifically for getting physical. Our ancestors didn't think about it because every single thing they did or had, was because of physical labor. They were actually challenged with looking for ways to make things less physical to give their body a break.

You can fit everyday activity in by taking brisk walks, gardening, biking, walking to the grocery store instead of driving, swimming and so forth. If you overdo it in the physical activity department you will stress your system, aging you faster and zapping your energy stores. Balance is the key and where there's a will there's a way.

My Thoughts . . .
Sometime we just need to stop and think logical. What our ancestors did and how they functioned physiologically makes sense. Their eating, sleeping and physical exercise patterns make sense, yet we often ignore them just because. If you are serious about your health you will find since in ways past and start applying.

Nutrients Your Body Needs

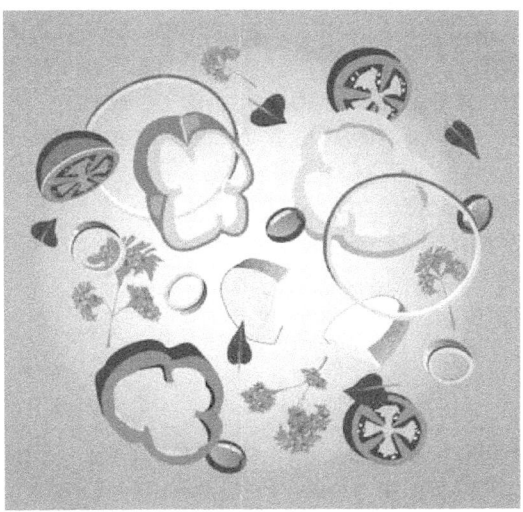

Your body is a finely tuned machine that needs to be fueled optimally long-term if you want it to perform better, keeping your healthy and disease free. The nutrients your body needs is non-negotiable, an absolute you either deliver or suffer the consequence. Using the knowledge you have and opening your mind to learning more healthy eating strategies, you are only going to make your body stronger and healthier and there is only good in that.

I don't want to overload you here because this is a introductory book, but it's important you are familiar with the main nutrients your body needs and why.

Lean Protein - Protein is an important part of every single cell in your body, including hair and nails that are mainly protein. Protein is used to repair and manufacture tissues, enzymes, hormones and numerous other internal chemicals. I'm sure you've heard protein is the building block of muscles, skin, cartilage, bones and blood too. This macronutrient, required in large doses, is not stored in the body like carbohydrates and fats, other macronutrients. Because of this it's critical you eat protein rich foods regularly for energy and optimal health. In general 2-3 servings of protein each day is adequate. Remembering a serving of meat is the size of a deck of cards.

Lean Protein Sources:
- Chicken breast
- Lean Beef
- Fish/Seafood
- Eggs
- Beans
- Nuts
* Milk and milk products are also a source of protein but is quite controversial as we've discussed.

Natural Complex Carbohydrates - Complex carbohydrates give your body long-term energy. Unfortunately they've been put through the ringer in recent times because they've been abused and used. Choosing to eat unhealthy simple carbs like white breads and pastas, muffins and pastries in excess, is going to cause weight gain and interfere with weight loss, steal energy and leave you feeling sluggish and depressed. There are two types of carbohydrates and your system wants complex for the most part.

SIMPLE CARBOHYDRATES - You'll find these in things like grapes, peaches, apples, milk, white breads, pasta, rice, cakes, pastries, candies and sweets. Simple natural carbohydrates that are found in fruits for example, are much healthier than processed options. Vitamins, minerals and fiber are found in natural simple carbohydrates like healthy fruits are good for your body. The processed option offers little or no nutritional value.

COMPLEX CARBOHYDRATES - Better known as starches, complex carbs give your body energy, lots of fiber and important vitamins and minerals. Natural carbo-hydrates are your best choice here.

Natural Complex Carb Sources:
- Oatmeal
- Oat bran and wheat germ
- Barley, Buckwheat and Cornmeal
- Yams, cauliflower, corn, carrots and onion
- Raw peas, spinach, turnip, asparagus, cabbage, cu-cumbers and celery
- Lentils, onions, and artichokes
- Beans and potatoes
* Whole grain breads/pastas/rice are good sources of complex carbohydrates sparingly because they are pro-cessed. A good portion of your caloric intake needs to come from complex carbohydrates so make sure you get at least 4-5 servings daily.

Good Fats (Unsaturated) - You need fat to survive and function. Unsaturated fats help protect your heart and support overall good health. Good fats like omega-3 fats-are critical to your emotional and physical well-being. Fat helps manage your moods, think more clearly, battle fatigue and keep your weight stable. Cutting fat out of your diet isn't the answer to getting healthy. It's all about making healthy fat choices in moderation and removing bad fats from your menu. Eating a healthy and well-balanced diet will naturally give you more than enough fat in most cases.

Good Fats Sources:
- Olive oil, canola oil and sunflower oil
- Sesame oil, avocados and olives

- Nuts and peanut butter
- Soybean oil, corn oil and safflower oil
- Sunflower seeds, sesame seeds and pumpkin seeds
- Fatty fish, tofu and soymilk

Bad Fats - Increases the risk of specific diseases and come in the form of saturated and Trans fat. Experts agree Trans fat is worse than saturated fat because is chemically altered fat found often in cakes and pastries to extend shelf life and decrease the cost of production.

Bad Fats Sources:
- High fat meats
- Butter and cheese
- Ice cream, lard and dairy products
- Coconut oil and palm oil
- Cakes, pastries, cookies, donuts and other packaged sweets
- Microwave popcorn and vegetable shortening
- Fried fast foods
- Chocolate bars

Ideally you need to keep your total caloric intake of "good" fats to under 35%, with less than 10% of that saturated.

NOTE- Coconut oil is a saturated oil, but is an exception to the rule because experts have found all sorts of health benefits from boosting immune system function to clearing up skin conditions and so much more.

Fiber
Fiber Sources:
- Beans and nuts
- Oatmeal
- Berries and vegetables
* Whole grains, brown rice and brown pasta sparingly.

Vitamins and Minerals - It doesn't have to be so hard! By eating a well balanced Perfect Health Diet you are going to get all the essential vitamins and minerals your body needs to thrive. Your body needs:

- Calcium - Bone growth, blood clotting, muscle contraction, nerve transmission
- Choline - Helps produce cells and neurotransmitters
- Chromium - Aids in controlling blood sugars
- Copper - Metabolism of iron
- Fiber - Digestion, purging of toxins, levels blood sugars
- Fluoride - Helps protect teeth, stimulates bone growth
- Folate - Essential in cell development, metabolism of protein, heart health and fetal development
- Iodine - Key in thyroid function
- Iron - Component of red blood cells
- Magnesium - Assists with heart rhythm, bone strength and nerves
- Manganese - Helps in bone formation
- Molybdenum - Production of enzymes
- Phosphorus - Helps cells function normally
- Potassium - Helps maintain fluid balance, control blood pressure
- Selenium - Regulate hormone and protects cells
- Sodium - Fluid balance
- Vitamin A - Vision, reproduction and immune function
- Thiamin - Processing of carbohydrates and protein
- Riboflavin - Helps in metabolism and making food energy
- Niacin - Cholesterol production and food energy
- Pantothenic Acid - Helps with fatty acid metabolism
- Vitamin B6 - Essential for nervous system and metabolizing sugars and protein
- Biotin - Synthesis of fats and amino acids
- Cobalamin - Helps produce red blood cells
- Vitamin C - Protects against cell damage, strengthens immunity, makes collagen

- Vitamin D - Helps metabolize calcium
- Vitamin E - Antioxidant protecting against cell damage
- Vitamin K - Blood clotting and bone health
- Zinc - Helps immunity, reproduction and nerve function
Essential Vitamins and minerals are found in a variety of healthy foods including fresh fruits and vegetables, eggs and nuts, lean meats, beans, seeds, fish and tea. The key is making sure you eat a diversified range of healthy foods so that you get all the vitamins and minerals your body needs and you will get this with The Perfect Health Diet.

My Thoughts . . .
Your body needs to be fueled properly, in the right amounts and on a regular basis in order to optimize your health. By making sure you get all the macro and micro-nutrients you need each day, energy will be plentiful, your weight will naturally fall into your "normal" range, and se-rious disease will be deterred instead of inevitable. You are important and this means it's time for you to imple-ment your Perfect Health Diet. It's important to figure out what "fits" for you.

Food Myths

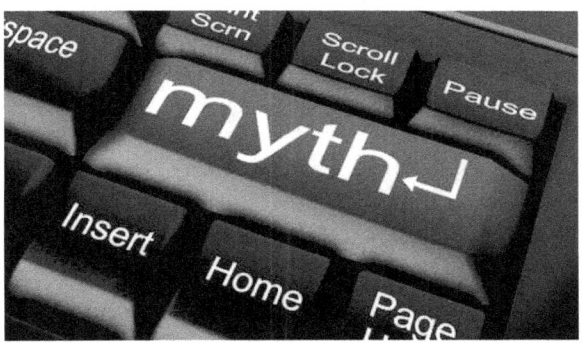

Most food and nutrition myths have at least a smidgeon of truth. Problem is you need "the whole truth and nothing but the truth" if you are going to succeed in creating your Perfect Health Diet thereby losing fat, strengthening muscles, decreasing aches and pains, gaining energy, boosting immune system function, sharpening thinking and tapping into optimism as a result.
By separating fact from fiction we'll debunk these Food Myths and arm you with effective ammo and not just blanks.

Tale 1 - Eggs will harm your heart
Truth -Yes eggs do contain a reasonable amount of cholesterol that under certain criteria can help block arteries in unhealthy people. Lucky for us experts agree an egg a day when eating healthy and exercising isn't a bad thing. It's the saturated and Trans fat found heavily in fried foods and packaged cakes, cookies, pies, donuts and other sweets that is going to feed your bad cholesterol level. On the flip side, eggs have healthy protein and iron that helps battle low energy and build your muscles strong.

As with everything, moderation is the key.

Tale 2 - Eating a raw food diet is necessary for smooth digestion

Truth - Raw foods are the ultimate in healthy because no nutrients are lost in the cooking process. What you see is what you get! Some experts claim eating raw food aids better digestion because the plant enzymes are pre-served. This claim isn't true because they aren't necessary for human health.

Tale 3 - Calories eaten in the evening turn right into fat

Truth - Calories are calories and it really doesn't matter when you eat them. That said, it makes sense to eat more calories for energy earlier in the day, assuming that's when you're most active. Your body will trust you more and burn more calories if you ensure the calories are available for utilization when required.

Tale 4 - Microwave radiation is dangerous for food

Truth - When you think of radiation you might think "nu-clear bomb." There's no need to worry here because a microwave cooks food from the inside out so nothing from the microwave alters the food negatively. Be sure you use microwave safe containers though, because the plastic may leak chemicals into the food in minute amounts otherwise.

Tale 5 - If you are missing key nutrients in your diet you will crave specific foods

Truth - Well cows love to lick blocks of blue salt when they need iodine, it's instinctive. As far as we know hu-man food cravings are learned and all about emotional eating. If a food is "taboo" we want it more. There is one exception to the rule here and that's iron. If lacking iron some people crave laundry soap, clay, and even cement. It's weird, but true.

Tale 6 - It's healthy to fast on a regular basis to remove toxins from your system
Truth - Just the same as ancient times back 2500 years ago, your body is crafted to naturally purge harmful toxins from interfering with your good health through the spleen, kidneys and liver. Experts agree that there is no evidence proving fasting or detoxing with juice works better.

Tale 7 - Salads are the healthy choice
Truth - Stop right there! It all depends on what sort of salad you are having and your thoughts on that oh-so-dangerous salad dressing. More often than not if you're having a little bit of lettuce with your salad dressing you are better off having a burger and fries - I kid you not. A healthy salad choice would be a spinach salad with fresh veggies, grilled chicken and a drizzle of salad dressing. By always ordering salad dressing on the side you have control of how much fat you're putting one. In basics, one tablespoon has a hundred calories of fat.

Tale 8 - It's always better to have fresh fruit
Truth - Dried fruit contains just as many nutrients as fresh fruit and stores longer, with the exception of Vitamin C. Not to mention just one tablespoon of dried fruit equals one whole serving of fresh fruit.

Tale 9 - Blood pressure is boosted by eating salt
Truth - This is a tall tale from the 40s. Studies show a person with normal blood pressure doesn't have to worry about decreasing their salt intake, although, if you have high blood pressure you're more likely to develop salt-sensitivity where you may benefit from keeping an eye on your salt intake. Take note it's actually potassium that's more critical to lowering blood pressure. So you should

increase your intake of broccoli, spinach, bananas and beans to help decrease your blood pressure naturally.

My Thoughts . . .
Food myths can really steer you in the wrong direction, which makes setting the record straight important. The more accurate information you get the better. The closer you will get to creating and using your Perfect Health Diet. You are important.

Best Energy Pick-Me-Ups

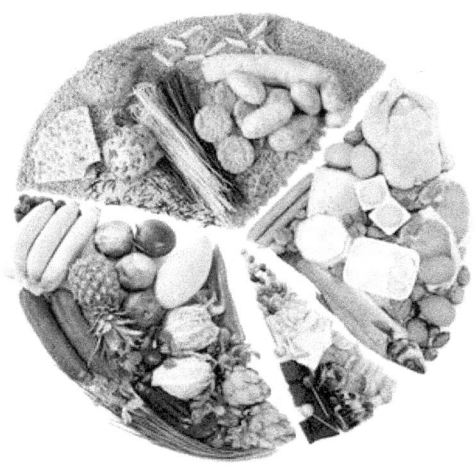

There are going to be times where you need a little bit of an energy boost. Maybe your tummy is rumbling or you didn't have time to finish all your lunch - it happens! Food energy is energy gained from food through cellular respiration, where oxygen attaches with food molecules in simple terms (aerobic respiration). The flip side is the shuffling of atoms in the molecules which is anaerobic respiration.

You need energy to function, to move your muscles, to think daily. Here are a few foods that will give you the zip you need fast.

Single Foods
Banana - Bananas are great energy boosts because they are quickly absorbed, full of energizing complex carbohy-

drates, potassium and loads of other vitamins and minerals.

Apple - They are a tasty and easy energy source that has slow-release energy. Meaning you are going to feel energized longer than many other simple carbs that spike your blood sugars and leave you drained faster than you can snap your fingers. Apples are also chalk full of healthy nutrients like potassium, Vitamin C and B, all of which are going to make your body very happy.

Berries - Fresh berries are excellent for energy. These sweet and tasty fruits are loaded with antioxidants that naturally protect your body from disease and illness. Add to that lots of essential vitamins and minerals your body needs to stay strong and you've got yourself a great snack choice.

Nuts - A handful of nuts is heading in the right direction when you're looking for fast energy. Almonds are full of great nutrients including Vitamin E, manganese, tryptophan, copper, magnesium, riboflavin and phosphorus. This great source of protein helps to protect your immune system, better sleep, relax muscles, alleviate stress AND boost immediate energy. Take note nuts are high in calories and good fats, so make sure you stop after a handful.

Peanut Butter - If you are in a pinch for time and need long-term energy fast, a tablespoon of peanut butter can do the trick. Loaded with protein and supporting nutrients your body needs to build muscle and stay strong, peanut butter is a smart choice.

Dried Fruit - This natural energy booster is going to give your body a nice boost of energy to burn. Full of good carbs and other vital nutrients to give you a boost, dried fruit is fast and easy to have around for snacking in a pinch.

Combination Foods

Often the best root to energize your body is combining foods, particularly lean protein and complex carbohydrates. This gives you the energy to build your body strong and keep your systems balanced and healthy, but also the staying power of the good carbs that will help you last longer than the Energizer Bunny that keeps going and going and going.

Peanut Butter and Celery - This snack gives your body access to quick long-lasting energy that gives you the full feeling because of the fibrous celery.

Grilled Chicken, Romaine and Spinach - Grabbing this out of the fridge is a quick and easy pick-me-up when you're on the run. Just grill a batch of chicken breasts beforehand and keep them in the fridge. All you do is wrap a piece of Romaine around the grilled chicken and add in some tasty powerful spinach. You get your vitamin C, calcium, protein and lots of other vital nutrients to boost you up fast.

Sweet Potato and Veggies - With a little bit of preparation you can get energized with something different. Just bake a couple sweet potatoes beforehand so they are still firm but tender. Slice them about 1/4 inch thick and mix them in with slice cucumbers, peppers, carrots and celery. This combo definitely packs a punch.

Fruit Cup - Throw together a dish of berries, pineapple, mango, pears, banana, oranges, and any other fruit you favor. You'll get a rich source of Vitamin C, thiamin, manganese, fiber, copper and B6 to start. Tasty and healthy, need I say more?

Medley of Beans - Beans are great energy boosters. Beans are considered in both the meat and vegetable groups. They are full of protein, complex carbohydrates and lots of other vitamins to keep your body healthy. Kidney beans, black beans, chickpeas, and lentils are just a few to experiment with. All you need to do is give them a cook, mix and eat up!

My Thoughts . . .
Planning is everything when you are looking to set yourself up for success in the eating department. By having healthy and energizing options to satiate hunger when it strikes, you are going to help curb cravings, reduce overeating and re-program your mind to cooperate with your body, both striving to build your body lean, healthy and strong. Don't be afraid to experiment and find the food combinations that fit best with your preferences and tolerances. If you can't eat happily it's just not going to last.

Food Tips to Lose Weight

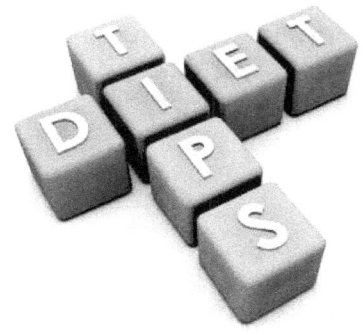

Losing weight for most of us isn't easy. If it was we'd like-ly all be walking around about the size of toothpicks. Unhealthy or not, that seems to be what those social stressing magazines dictate these days, societal pres-sures that are both unrealistic and deadly dangerous, particularly on young girls.

What's important here is that you do what's right for you. Pay attention to your preference and tolerances and un-derstand that what works for one person might not do the same for you. That's perfectly okay because all you've got to do is make the minor adjustments necessary, in a healthful light, to find the "fit" for you and your lifestyle.

Make food changes that are positive and manageable for you long term. If you can't make your food changes last for the long haul, then you might as well not even bother. Perspective is what you need to keep in mind. Here are a few food pointers that will help you take advantage of the factors you can control, setting yourself up for weight loss success and a much healthier you.

* **Slow Down** - We always seem to be running a hundred miles a minute in today's world. Half the time, we are wolfing down food and not even tasting what we're eating. Shame on us! Practice consciously stopping yourself and pay attention to what you are eating. Things about how it tastes, feels in your mouth, chew slowly and actual "enjoy" the flavors. This will help you get eat less and get more satisfaction.

* **Plan Ahead** - Planning your meals ahead is going to help you with long-term gain. If you are serious about creating your Perfect Health Diet you are going to have to think ahead. This will also help divert dangerous habits of yesteryear from popping up. If you know you are going to have a tasty grilled chicken salad when going out with the girls, you'll be less likely to order your traditionally chicken wings and fries. It's all about making the decision to make positive eating changes in your life and making them happen. If you know what you are eating for the week you can have some of it prepared beforehand and this may help to alleviate snacking while you are thinking about what you're going to eat and then again when you are actually preparing it.

* **Portion Sizes** - It's so very critical that you know your portion sizes. For instance when eating out at a restaurant I can pretty much guarantee you're going to get a serving that's at least twice the amount your body needs. The solution is to package half your meal up in a doggy bag before you even take a bite. This way you aren't going to overeat and you will have lunch or dinner ready for the next day! Understand basic portion sizes to help teach your body that it really doesn't need to eat a whole chicken to be full.

Meat = about the size of a deck of cards or 4 oz
Potatoes = 1/2 - 3/4 cup
Veggies = 1 cup
Oatmeal (cooked) = 3/4 cup
Oil/fats = 1 tablespoon
Salad Dressing = 1-2 tablespoons (sparingly)
Whole Grain Bread (on occasion) = 1 slice
Whole Grain Bagel (on occasion) = 1/2 bagel
Whole Grain Rice/Pasta (on occasion) = 1/2-3/4 cup

Facts for Thought - Without water no life would exist. Without it you would die within a few days. Your brain is 95% water, lungs 90% and blood 82%. In fact your body is about 2/3rds liquid energy. Water helps regulate your internal body temperature, lubricate your intricate bodily systems so they can function optimally, flushes harmful toxins and transports essential nutrients throughout your body.
Hydrating your body with 6-8 glasses a day will do your body very well. Of course you will need to replenish these stores if you happen to be exercising heavily or live in a warmer climate than most.

My Thoughts . . .
Getting healthy and losing weight is not a black and white issue. There are so many affective factors involved that you need to learn through trial and error what works and what doesn't for you. It's all about taking the food information you are gathering and twist and tweak it so it helps you in health. There is no "right" or "wrong" here, just better. Take the food strategies here that are applicable for you and get "better."

Processed Food 101- It Kills!

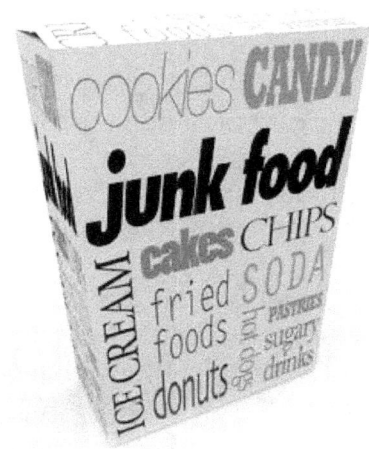

We are surrounded by processed foods. Walking down the grocery store isles you see a melody of beautifully packaged foods that seem magnetic. Something so wonderfully inviting has to be healthy for you right? WRONG! *What is Processed Food?*

Processed food isn't just what you get from a fast food joint. It's also . . .

* Foods that are boxed, packaged, jarred or canned, with a whole whack of ingredients on the label, many of which you can't even pronounce.

* Refrigerated, frozen, canned, and dehydrated foods. These foods have been taken from their natural and healthy state to be "chemical-ized." This helps manufac-

turers make more money and you get to keep them longer before they spoil, if they ever do.

Processing is all about convenience and food manufac-
turers love to add a few extras in while they are at it.
There are a few extra ingredients processed foods are
subject to for specific purposes:

- Stabilization so that your soup doesn't separate
- Texturizing so your cereal doesn't get mushy
- Coloring so your food looks yummy
- Flavoring so that food items taste "new and improved"
- Preserving so you can enjoy these processed foods for
years to come
- Bleaching helps to disinfect and deodorize
- Sweeteners to change the flavor to favorable
- Emulsifiers so that oils and water will stay mixed
- Odor eaters to make sure you can smell all the crap in
processed foods
Processed Foods Can . . .
* Cause cancer
* Increase the risk of obesity
* Contribute to heart disease and stroke
* Cause extreme fluctuations in blood sugars, leading to
serious disease like diabetes
* Make your body less efficient in absorbing required nu-
trients
* Fill your body with harmful toxins that interfere with in-
ternal system function
* Zap energy and trigger nasty mood swings
Unfortunately today we live in a world where convenience
and money take precedence over good health and opti-
mal lifestyle choices. Here are some common processed
foods to steer clear of in for the sake of good health.

Processed Foods to Steer Clear Of . . .
- Bologna and other packaged luncheon meats

- Hot dogs, sausage and bacon
- Fruits and vegetables that are canned (frozen is fine)
- White rice, pasta and bread
- Cookies, chips, crackers, cakes and pastries
- Boxed lunches like macaroni and hamburger helper
- Boxed sides like stuffing, scalloped and mashed potatoes
- Canned pastas like spaghetti and ravioli
- Frozen dinners, fish sticks, chicken sticks, burgers and French fries
- Ice cream and ice cream cakes
- Frozen or refrigerated pre-made baking, like cookies and rolls

The idea here is to make food choices that are natural and wholesome. Things that are natural and not filled with dangerous chemicals and preservative to make them last longer. Sure a nice piece of lean grilled steak is good for you. But if you buy some pre-packaged meat that's good in the fridge for a weak, isn't that signaling you with a bright red danger flag? Natural doesn't last, it spoils fast. A good thing because this means you aren't loading your body with non-nutrient items that are toxic, particularly in large quantities over time, which is EXACTLY what processed foods will do to your body. They will poison it.

My Thoughts . . .
Our society is conditioned to look favorably on processed foods without a second guess. The time has come to start paying attention to the food choices going into your body and to make better ones. Your Perfect Health Diet is going to make a huge positive impact on your life. But if this is going to happen for the most part you're going to have to kiss processed foods good-bye. It's a choice you have to make. Do it or don't but I don't want to hear you whining about it in the meantime.

Top Foods to Avoid

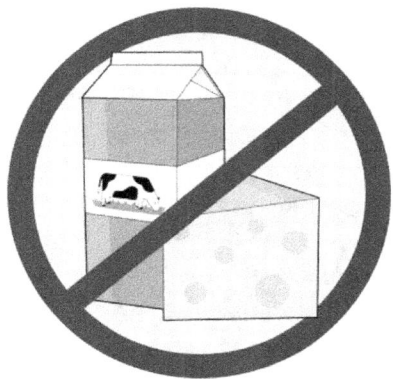

Some foods have a nastier bite than others. Here are a few of the top offenders to run away from.

FRENCH FRIES - I'm so sorry but French fries are one of those foods you are best not to bother with. These cleverly disguised potatoes are full of bad oil, fat and sodium, and have lost almost all nutrients in the overcooking process.

HEALTHY ALTERNATIVE - Baked sweet potato fries. Cut up a sweet potato, brush lightly with healthy safflower or olive oil, sprinkle with fresh herbs and bake. I think these are even tastier than their cousin and a heck of a lot healthier!

DONUTS/CAKES - Donuts are just fried cake better and you aren't getting any healthy nutrients from them. Just loads of unhealthy fat and calories.

HEALTHY ALTERNATIVE - Better than a donut for a treat is an all-natural rice cake smeared with peanut butter, or three for that matter! A couple of whole grain crackers naked, works too. If you need some sweetness you can always drizzle a touch of natural honey atop.

CHIPS - Have you ever wondered how many pounds of chips you chow down in a year? Chips have nothing healthy about them. They just serve up a nice dose of fat, oil and salt to bung your health up and make you thirsty for more sugar laden soda.

HEALTHY ALTERNATIVE - A handful of mixed nuts works well. This will satisfy your salt craving and give you a nutrient dense snack that will keep your belly full longer.

SODA - Talk about spiking your blood sugar levels. You might as well just drink a cup of sugar and avoid some of the added chemicals.

HEALTHY ALTERNATIVE - All natural flavored mineral water is fabulous. Experiment with your favored fruits and herbs, combine them with filtered water and leave overnight. Now you'll have a tasty and healthy vitamin rich beverage that NEVER gets boring.

FROZEN DINNERS - Most frozen dinners "look" healthy but are anything but. Packed with saturated fat and sodium that will make your heart stop cold. Even the veggies are often so overcooked they have very little nutritional value when all is said and done.

HEALTHY ALTERNATIVE - Take the time to cook your own meals. With a little planning it really doesn't take very much time at all. By picking a day to slice up your veggies for the weak and grill or broil up any meats you are going to enjoy you can make is so that you literally walk in the door, toss the ingredients together, warm up and enjoy.

My Thoughts . . .
It's a start anyway. Knowing what foods to stay away from is just as important and so is understanding which foods are best for you. Don't expect yourself to be perfect here. Just recognize that each positive move you make will better you physically, mentally and emotionally, bringing you another step closer to your Perfect Health Diet.

Healthful Diet Plan

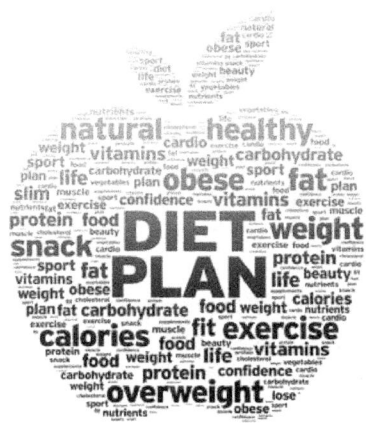

Here's where you need to take what you know about you, your preferences and tolerances, the information you have added here to your arsenal, and your common sense if figure out healthier eating. Your job is to connect the dot because there are so many variables to consider before you can fine tune your Perfect Health Diet.

For example, here are a few of the basics that are going to alter the amount of calories you consume each day in order to provide for your body, keep your energy levels up and drop fat:

* Height and weight
* Activity level
* Body composition
* Genetics
* Medical conditions/overall health
* Lifestyle

* Metabolic rate

To start what you need to do is establish a base level eating strategy from which to build. There are even calculators on-line that can give you an idea of how many calories you need eat each day by plugging in your height, weight and activity level (BMI). It's a great place from which to start.

To give you an idea, the average woman needs about 2000 calories a day to maintain her weight. In order to lose weight she can lower the number of calories eaten, increase activity level or both. Men on average need about 2400 calories each day to keep their weight steady This is all dependant on preferences and tolerances and how committed you are to getting healthier. I can give you all the detailed scientific stats you need but if you aren't going to apply it then it means "diddly" squat! Let it be YOUR CHOICE!

Times have changed in lifestyle in the past 2500 years somewhat drastically. Lower is the quality of foods available to us because of how our foods are prepared and delivered and economics. Organic foods that are the healthier choice are more costly. Some just can't afford this option. Over time some argue it's more beneficial to focus the majority of calories on fresh fruits and vegetables. This will help flush more harmful toxins out of your system that have built up over time, while providing more readily available nutrients for your system to utilize. Not to mention the fact that plant sources like soy, hempseeds and chlorella, a type of single cell green algae, are great sources of protein. The most important factor here is realizing a large chunk of your diet should come from lean meats and vegetables, followed by fruits and then natural grains minimally. Fats of course are used sparingly and ensure they are healthy unsaturated fats.

Eating Strategy Guidelines
WOMEN 2000 cal/day
* 3-4 servings - Lean meats and meat alternatives -fish, eggs, beef, lamb, chicken, duck, shellfish and fatty fish (shoot for at least 2 servings of fatty fish per week)
* 5-6 servings of carbohydrates - vegetables, beans, nuts, natural grains in moderation, fruits in moderation
* 1-2 servings of healthy fats - olive oil, avocado, safflower oil etc.

SAMPLE DAY EATING 3 TIMES - Similar to our ancestors
Meal 1
- Eggs (2 boiled) 100-150 cal
- Vegetables (1 cup cooked spinach) 100-150 cal
- Fruit (banana, 1 cup berries) 100-150 cal
Meal 2 (Grilled Chicken Salad)
- 1 grilled chicken breast 150-200 cal
- 2 cups Romaine lettuce (celery, cucumber, tomato, carrots, sprouts) 100-200 cal
- 1/2 cup nuts 150-200 cal
- 1 cup kidney beans 100-150 cal
- 1 cup fresh fruit 100-150 cal
- 1-2 tablespoons oil dressing 100-200 cal
Meal 3 - Broiled Salmon
- 1 serving salmon broiled with herbs and spices, drizzle of olive oil 200-300 cal
- 2 cups streamed vegetables (broccoli, cauliflower, Brussels sprouts) 200-250 cal
- 1/2 cup quinoa 100-150 cal

My Thoughts . . .
This is just a sample of the type of eating that's going to help your body fill up with vital nutrients and purge all the

toxins built up. In time you will learn how to alternate foods and make food swaps that work for you. Keep an open mind here and realize the first step is to plant the idea of change into your head and to give you the basics to visualize it happening. Get used to the idea, experiment and configure the information you've gathered to make it your Perfect Health Diet.

The Physical Matters

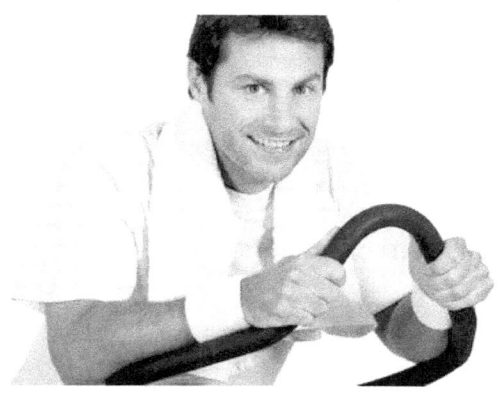

Here we go back to the days of the cave man, but it is important to show you just how important regular daily physical activity is in your life. This doesn't mean you are going to have to train for 2-3 hours at the gym each day, or join a running club that meets daily to literally run you through the ringer. This means that you need to figure out what sort of physical activities you enjoy and make sure you prioritize this and make it happen regularly.

I'm not here to lecture you about physical activity or go into detail about it. All I want is to ensure you understand if you want the Perfect Health Diet for you. To lose fat, get healthy and keep it off, then you are going to have to get your body moving too. The hardest part is the first step and if you can do that and keep up with it for about 6 weeks it will turn into a healthy new habit, one that you won't have to think about and it's only going to help you get healthy for life and feel fantastic about it, mentally and physically.

Benefits of Exercising Regularly

* Burns fat by increasing metabolic rate
* Increases circulation which helps internal systems function optimally
* Releases natural endorphins, chemicals that make you "feel good"
* Increases energy
* Improves cognitive capacity
* Flips your perspective to positive
* Helps improve sleep
* Combats health conditions and disease

Beginner Plan
* 30-45 minutes cardiovascular activity per day (hiking, biking, swimming, running, gardening, fast walking, aerobics, treadmill, tennis)
* 15-20 minutes strength training/weights 2-3 days per week (getting started with a personal trainer is your best option to ensure you are performing each exercise correctly and avoid injury)

My Thoughts . . .
The most important factor here is that you open your mind to exercising regularly, that you get into a routine and stick with it. Diversity is the key to getting results so make certain you change things up regularly. Test the waters and try different activities until you find the one that "fits" for you.
If you don't like being stuck in the gym you can try an outdoor boot camp training session or join a biking group with your friends. Some people are happy having a few pieces of cardiovascular equipment at home with some weights. Consider your tolerances and preferences and make sure you follow your gut and NEVER give up.
Sure you don't have to get physical for survival like your ancestors, but this doesn't mean your body doesn't need

strenuous exercise. By this I mean exercise that makes you sweat, because going through the motions is just kidding yourself.
You can do it I know you can, one step at a time and always check with your doctor first to be safe.

Final Thoughts

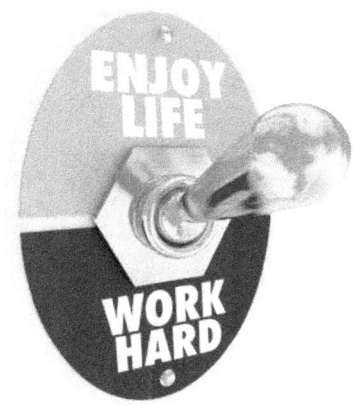

Your Perfect Health Diet is a huge step in the right direction and you should be proud of taking the first step. Life is extremely precious and unfortunately as humans we tend to take things for granted until they are gone. Your health is something you don't want to fool with because once it's gone you can't have it back in most instances.

By fueling your body "right," with plenty of lean protein, good carbohydrates and healthy fats, combined with regular exercise, you are going to build your mind and body strong and they will work united to make you a better you. Helping to fight off disease, avoid injury and recover from illness and disease faster, all while feeling energetic and alive, excited to tackle the next life challenge.

You deserve to be healthy, happy and strong and your Perfect Health Diet is the tool to get you there. This isn't a fad diet or temporary change in your life. If you are serious about your health and wellness your Perfect Health Diet is a concept of healthy change. With numerous controllable health adjustments you need to make and keep so that a long and adventurous life is what you will have ahead of you.

Open your mind, keep learning about healthy life choices and make adjustments along the way that work for you. Be able to forgive yourself when you step backwards, recognize this, be okay with it and pick right back up on the right path. The one that is going to leave you feeling great about yourself and looking slimmer and trimmer for bonus points.

The ball's in your court, it's time for you to take some serious action, work hard and reap the rewards.

We have the choice to look for the positive or the negative in life. You can choose to lift someone up or to stomp on them. Writing is my passion and I work hard at it, with the goal of helping make people better. If you gain a new piece of knowledge, read something that makes you think, or perhaps even smile a few times, then I am happy and content!

Life's just too short not to tune into optimism. If your glass is half full, then I invite you to read my writing, and if you have a minute to spare when you're through, **I would appreciate your review.** This will help me better myself and my writing. I thank you in advance and appreciate you.

www.ingramcontent.com/pod-product-compliance
Lightning Source LLC
Chambersburg PA
CBHW071122280526
45787CB00003B/1137